Table of Contents

PREVIEW

Acid reflux is what happens when some of the acid content of the stomach flows up into the esophagus. Heartburn is the burning feeling a person gets when they have acid reflux. Frequent acid reflux may mean a person has GERD.

Although people may use the terms interchangeably, heartburn is a symptom of acid reflux, also known Trusted Source as gastroesophageal reflux (GER). Despite the name, heartburn has nothing to do with the heart.

Gastroesophageal reflux disease (GERD) is a more serious form of GER. Doctors will diagnose GERD when acid reflux becomes a recurrent complaint about an individual, usually more than twice a weekTrusted Source for several weeks at a time.

GERD is most common in Western countries, affecting an estimated 20%Trusted Source of the population in these regions.

About 20% of Americans also have GERD, and it is the most commonTrusted Source gastrointestinal condition diagnosed in the outpatient setting.

About 60% of people who have GERD are women. Among people living with GERD, African Americans account for the second-largest group after people who are white.

ACID REFLUX DIET RECIPES

BREAKFAST

1. Cheeseburger Pasta

Prep Time: 25 Minutes

Cook Time: 60 Minutes

Servings: 4

Ingredients

- 1 medium onion (quartered)
- 8 ounces mushrooms (quartered)
- 1 small zucchini (cut into 1 inch chunks)
- 1 Tbsp. olive oil
- 12 ounces 95/5 ground beef
- 2 Tbsp. no salt added tomato paste
- 1/2 tsp. salt
- black pepper to taste
- 1 tsp. paprika
- 2 tsp. garlic powder

- 1 cup no salt added vegetable stock
- 1 cup 2% milk
- 1 cup elbow pasta
- 1 ounce reduced fat cheddar cheese (shredded)
- 2 Tbsp. reduced fat sour cream

Instructions

1. Place the onion in a food processor fitted with a chopping blade and pulse until they are the size of small dice. Set aside.
2. Add the mushrooms to the food processor and pulse until they are the size of a small dice. Set aside.
3. Add the zucchini to the food processor and pulse until they are the size of a large dice.
4. Set aside.
5. Place the olive oil in a large skillet over high heat.
6. Add the onion and cook for 2 minutes. Stir frequently.
7. Add the mushrooms and cook for 5 minutes. Stir frequently.
8. Add the zucchini and cook for 5 minutes until most of the liquid has evaporated. Stir frequently and adjust the heat so the vegetables do not burn.

9. Add the ground beef and cook for about 4 to 5 minutes until browned.

10. Add the tomato paste, salt, pepper, paprika garlic powder, vegetable stock, milk, and pasta to the pan.

11. Stir and cover the pan.

12. Adjust the heat to a simmer.

13. Cook for 10 to 15 minutes until the pasta is just tender. Stir occasionally.

14. Uncover, stir, and simmer for two minutes.

15. Remove from the heat and stir in the cheddar cheese and sour cream.

16. Serve.

Prep Time: 50 Minutes

Cook Time: 3hrs 30 Minutes

Servings: 8

Ingredients

- 4 cloves garlic (minced)
- 1 small red onion (minced)
- 1 Tbsp ground cumin
- 2 tsp dried oregano
- 1/2 tsp salt
- fresh ground black pepper to taste
- 4 cups no salt added chicken broth (divided)
- 1 lime (juiced)
- 1 Tbsp no salt added tomato paste
- 1/4 cup apple cider vinegar
- 1 chipotle in adobo (left whole)
- 1 dried ancho chile (left whole)
- 2 lbs beef chuck (trimmed of excess fat)

Instructions

1. Preheat the oven to 300F.

   Add the garlic, onion, cumin, oregano, salt, pepper, 1

cup chicken broth, lime juice, tomato paste, vinegar, chipotle, ancho and beef to a large pot or dutch oven fitted with a lid.

Cover and place the pot in the oven. Cook for 5 hours. Add 1 cup of chicken broth after each of the 2nd, 3rd and 4th hours. Stir well after each time you add the chicken broth.

Remove the meat to a cutting board to cool.

2. Allow the braising liquid to cool somewhat, then puree until smooth.

Using a fork or pair of tongs, pull the beef apart along the grain. Place the pulled beef in a bowl and add the pureed sauce. Mix thoroughly.

Prep Time: 10 Minutes

Cook Time: 30 Minutes

Servings: 2

Ingredients

- 1/2 tsp olive oil
- 1/4 poblano chili (seeded and diced)
- 1 ear corn (shave kernels from the cob)
- 2 green onions (sliced crosswise)
- 1/2 medium red bell pepper (seeded and julienned)
- 1/4 tsp ground cumin
- 1 tsp chili powder
- 1/8 tsp salt
- fresh ground black pepper to taste
- 1/2 cup water
- 2 Tbsp fresh cilantro leaves (chopped)
- spray oil
- 4 corn tortillas
- 2 ounces Monterey jack cheese (shredded)

Instructions

1. Heat the olive oil in a large skillet over medium heat and add the poblano. Cook for about 3 minutes until slightly soft.

    Add the corn and increase the heat to medium-high. Cook the corn kernels, tossing frequently, until they begin to brown.

    Add the green onions and red pepper and cook for about 3 minutes.

    Add the cumin, chili powder, salt, pepper and cook for 2 minutes stirring continuously.

    Add the water and cook for about 7 to 10 minutes. Stir occasionally.

    When the water is evaporated, turn off the heat and add the cilantro. Toss until blended into the vegetable mixture.

    Preheat a non-stick griddle or pan over medium-high heat.

    After it is hot, spray lightly with oil and place 2 corn tortillas in the pan.

    Top each tortilla with the 1/4 of the cheese and then 1/2 of the corn mixture. Top the corn mixture with the remaining cheese.

Place another tortilla on top of the corn and cheese, forming the quesadilla. Spray very lightly with oil.

Cook for about 5 minutes on each side, pressing down to allow the cheese to melt into the corn, holding the quesadilla together. Turn at least once.

4. Chicken Piccata

Prep Time: 25 Minutes

Cook Time: 55 Minutes

Servings: 2

Ingredients

- 2 Tbsp. all-purpose flour or garbanzo flour
- 1/4 tsp. ground black pepper
- 2 tsp. extra virgin olive oil
- 1 tsp. unsalted butter
- 8 ounces boneless, skinless chicken breast
- 1/4 cup no salt added chicken or vegetable stock
- 2 Tbsp. white wine
- 4 tsp. capers
- 1/2 lemon (juiced)
- 1/2 tsp. lemon zest
- 1/8 tsp. salt
- 1/4 tsp. sugar

Instructions

1. Preheat the oven to 200°F.

2. Using a very sharp knife, carefully slice chicken breast on the bias into 1/2 inch thick slices (meat cut this way is called scaloppini).
3. Place the scaloppini between two sheets of plastic wrap and pound until they are about 1/4 inch thick.
4. Place the flour and pepper on a plate.
5. Place the chicken scaloppini in the flour and coat well.
6. Put the olive oil and butter in a large skillet over medium high heat and add the garlic.
7. Cook for about 2 minutes, and as the garlic begins to turn brown, add the chicken and cook for about 4 minutes on each side until browned on both sides.
8. Remove the chicken to a plate and place in the warm oven.
9. Add the chicken stock, white wine, lemon juice, lemon zest, capers, salt, and sugar to the pan and cook over medium heat, scraping the bottom of the pan until it is clean.
10. Cook for about 3 to 5 minutes until the flavor of alcohol has disappeared.
11. Add the chicken back into the pan for about 4 minutes, turning frequently.
12. The sauce will thicken to a glaze.
13. Place the chicken on a plate and top with the sauce.

Prep Time: 25 Minutes

Cook Time: 30 Minutes

Servings: 2

Ingredients

- 2 tsp. smoked paprika
- 1/8 tsp. salt
- 1/4 tsp. onion powder
- 1/4 tsp. garlic powder
- 1/4 tsp. cayenne pepper
- 1/4 tsp. fresh ground black pepper
- 1/4 tsp. dried thyme leaves
- 1/4 tsp. dried oregano leaves
- 2 4-ounce filets fresh red snapper
- 2 tsp. olive oil

Instructions

1. Place a skillet in the oven and preheat to 400°F.
2. Combine the paprika, salt, onion powder, garlic powder, cayenne pepper, black pepper, thyme, and oregano in a medium sized bowl.

3. Mix together until well blended.

4. Place the filets in the bowl and turn gently to coat the fish well with the spice mixture.

5. When the pan is hot, add the olive oil and swirl to coat the pan.

6. Place the fish in the hot pan skin side up and return the pan to the oven.

7. Cook for about 5 minutes and turn.

8. Cook for another 4 to 5 minutes and serve.

6. Chicken Fajitas with Roasted Red Peppers

Prep Time: 15 Minutes

Cook Time: 45 Minutes

Servings: 4

Ingredients

- 1 medium white onion (peeled and sliced thin)
- 1 quart water with ice
- 1 red bell pepper
- spray olive oil
- 12 ounces boneless skinless chicken breast (slice into thin strips)
- 1/4 tsp salt
- 1/4 tsp ground cumin
- 1/4 cup water
- 8 soft corn tortillas
- 2 tsp non-fat sour cream (per serving) (optional)
- 1 Tbsp fresh cilantro leaves (per serving)

Instructions

1. Place the sliced onion in a large mixing bowl and cover with the water and ice.

Preheat the oven to 350°F. Place the red pepper in the oven and roast for about 40 minutes. Turn the pepper a quarter turn about every ten minutes so that it roasts evenly. Remove the roasted pepper from the oven and place in a paper bag, closing the top. Allow the pepper to cool.

Once cool the skin of the pepper will slip off easily. Remove the seeds and slice the pepper very thin.

Heat a large non-stick skillet over medium-high heat. Once the pan is hot, drain the onions and add them to the pan. Stir frequently. As the excess water begins to evaporate, spray lightly with the olive oil.

2. Continue to cook until the onions are completely brown. If they cook too fast, reduce the heat to keep them from burning.

When the onions are well browned and limp, add the sliced roasted red bell pepper. Stir and increase the heat to medium-high and add the chicken, salt and cumin. Cook until the outside of the chicken strips are slightly browned.

Place a second skillet on another burner over high heat.

Add the water to the pan with the chicken mixture and cook, stirring frequently. The water will evaporate quickly and when there is only about a tablespoon left, remove the pan from the burner.

Place a tortilla in the second heated pan for about 5 - 10 seconds, turning once so that the tortilla is soft. Remove and repeat with a second tortilla. Layer the two corn tortillas together and fill with 1/4 of the fajita mixture, top with 2 teaspoons non-fat sour cream (optional) and 1 tablespoon cilantro leaves.

3. Repeat for the other three fajitas and serve.

Prep Time: 20 Minutes

Cook Time: 45 Minutes

Servings: 2

Ingredients

- 16 ounces boneless, skinless chicken thighs (cubed)
- 1 tsp. ground black pepper
- 2 lbs. onions (thinly sliced)
- 1 tsp. lemon zest
- 1/2 lemon (juiced)
- 1/4 tsp. salt
- 1/4 cup white wine
- 1 cup no salt added vegetable stock

Instructions

1. Place a small stock pot or medium dutch oven in the oven and preheat to 400°F.
2. When the pan is hot, remove and place over high heat.
3. Add the chicken thighs and cook for about 3 minutes.

4. Turn frequently, and when the chicken thighs are lightly browned, add the black pepper and onions.

5. Cook for another 4 minutes. Toss frequently.

6. Add the lemon zest, lemon juice, salt, white wine, and vegetable stock.

7. Stir and cover.

8. Place the covered pot in the oven and cook for 15 minutes.

9. Remove from the oven, stir gently and return to the oven uncovered.

10. Braise uncovered for another 20 minutes.

11. Serve.

Prep Time: 20 Minutes

Cook Time: 45 Minutes

Servings: 2

Ingredients

- 1/2 tsp. ground cumin
- 1 tsp. chili powder
- 1/2 tsp garlic powder
- 1/2 tsp onion powder
- To taste black pepper
- 1/4 tsp salt (divided)
- 1 head broccoli (cut into small florets)
- 1 bunch cauliflower (cut into small florets)
- 1 small red onion (thinly sliced)
- 4 tsp. olive oil
- 1 lb. boneless, skinless chicken thighs
- 1 Tbsp. no salt added tomato paste
- 1/2 tsp dried oregano
- 1 tsp. smoked paprika

Instructions

1. Preheat the oven to 350°F.
2. Line a baking sheet with aluminum foil.
3. Place the cumin, chili powder, garlic powder, onion power, pepper, and 1/8 teaspoon of the salt in a large bowl and mix well.
4. Toss broccoli, cauliflower and red onion with the seasoning blend and 2 teaspoons of the olive oil.
5. Place on the prepared baking sheet. Leave room for the chicken, it will be cooked on the same pan.
6. Place the remaining 2 teaspoons of olive oil in a small bowl with the tomato paste, oregano, smoked paprika, and 1/8 teaspoon of the salt.
7. Whisk well.
8. Add the whole chicken thighs to the bowl and toss to coat well.
9. Place the chicken thighs on the baking sheet with the vegetables.
10. Place the baking sheet in the oven.
11. Roast for about 12 to 15 minutes until the chicken reaches an internal temperature of 160° F. Toss the vegetables at least twice.
12. Allow chicken to rest for 3 to 5 minutes before serving.

Prep Time: 20 Minutes

Cook Time: 50 Minutes

Servings: 8

Ingredients

- 2 quarts water
- 2 tsp. white wine vinegar
- 12 ounces boneless, skinless chicken thighs
- 2 jalapeno peppers
- 1 cup cilantro
- 2 cloves garlic
- 2 Tbsp. reduced fat mayonnaise
- 1/4 cup reduced fat sour cream
- 1 Tbsp. olive oil
- 1/2 lime (juiced)
- 1 tsp. lime zest
- 1/4 tsp. salt
- 4 large ribs celery (cut into small dice)
- 4 large green onions (thinly sliced crosswise)

Instructions

1. Place the water and vinegar in a large skillet over medium high heat.
2. When water is almost boiling add the chicken thighs and cook for 10 to 15 minutes.
3. Remove, let cool for about 20 minutes and place in the refrigerator to chill.
4. Place the peppers, cilantro, garlic, mayonnaise, sour cream, olive oil, lime juice, lime zest, salt and fresh ground black pepper to taste in a blender and puree until smooth.
5. Place in the refrigerator to chill.
6. When the dressing and the chicken are chilled cut the chicken into 1/4 inch dice.
7. Place the chicken and the dressing in a bowl along with the celery and green onions.
8. Fold together well.
9. Serve.

Prep Time: 20 Minutes

Cook Time: 45 Minutes

Servings: 2

Ingredients

- 2 quarts water
- 2 tsp. white wine vinegar
- 12 ounces boneless, skinless chicken thighs
- 2 jalapeno peppers
- 1 cup cilantro
- 2 cloves garlic
- 2 Tbsp. reduced fat mayonnaise
- 1/4 cup reduced fat sour cream
- 1 Tbsp. olive oil
- 1/2 lime (juiced)
- 1 tsp. lime zest
- 1/4 tsp. salt
- 4 large ribs celery (cut into small dice)
- 4 large green onions (thinly sliced crosswise)
- 12 corn tortillas
- avocado (sliced)

Instructions

1   Place the water and vinegar in a large skillet over medium high heat.
2   When water is almost boiling add the chicken thighs and cook for 10 to 15 minutes.
3   Remove, let cool for about 20 minutes and place in the refrigerator to chill.
4   Place the peppers, cilantro, garlic, mayonnaise, sour cream, olive oil, lime juice, lime zest, salt and fresh ground black pepper to taste in a blender and puree until smooth.
5   Place in the refrigerator to chill.
6   When the dressing and the chicken are chilled cut the chicken into 1/4 inch dice.
7   Place the chicken and the dressing in a bowl along with the celery and green onions.
8   Fold together well.
9   Chill.
10 Place a large skillet or griddle over high heat.
11 When hot add tortillas three at a time and toast for about 3 to 5 minutes on each side.
12 When the tortillas are hot and slightly crispy fill with chicken salad and sliced avocado.
13 Serve.

LUNCH

Prep Time: 35 Minutes

Cook Time: 60 Minutes

Servings: 4

Ingredients

- 6 Tbsp. all purpose flour or garbanzo flour
- 2 tsp. olive oil
- 1 large onion (diced)
- 4 cloves garlic (minced)
- 2 large ribs celery (diced)
- 1 large green bell pepper (diced)
- 1 large red bell pepper (diced)
- 2 cup s no salt added vegetable stock
- 1 cup water
- 1/2 tsp. salt
- 1/4 tsp. freshly ground black pepper
- 1/8 tsp. cayenne
- 2 bay leaves

- 2 tsp. no salt added Cajun spice blend
- 1 15-ounce can no salt added diced tomatoes
- 2 Tbsp. dry sherry, or dry white wine
- 2 Tbsp. fresh parsley (chopped)
- 2 tsp. fresh thyme (chopped)
- 1 lb. shrimp, peeled and deveined
- 2 large green onions (thinly sliced crosswise)

Instructions

1. Place the flour in a large non-stick skillet and heat over medium-high heat.
2. Watch the pan carefully, stirring and shaking the flour. It will take about 10 to 15 minutes and the flour will turn an almond brown. Adjust the heat so that the flour does not cook too fast or burn. Remove to a plate and allow to cool.
3. Place the olive oil in the pan over medium heat, and add the diced onion.
4. Cook for about 3 minutes. Stir frequently.
5. Add the garlic and celery. Cook for about 2 minutes. Stir frequently.
6. Add the green and red peppers and cook for about 2 minutes.

7   Sprinkle about 1/4 of the cooked flour over the top of the cooked vegetables.

8   Stir to blend the flour and repeat with the flour in three more batches until it is fully incorporated and there are no clumps of flour.

9   Add the vegetable stock and water slowly stirring continuously.

10   As the sauce begins to thicken add the salt, pepper, cayenne pepper, bay leaf and Cajun spice.

11   Cook over medium low heat adding water a tablespoon at a time if the sauce is too thick.

12   Add the tomatoes, sherry, parsley and thyme. The sauce can be made to this point and kept warm or overnight.

13   When ready to serve heat the sauce and add the shrimp. Cook for about 8 to 10 minutes until they are pink and firm.

14   Serve over Brown Rice and top with the chopped green onions.

15   Note that the Nutrition Facts are for the Etouffee without the rice.

12. Salmon and Butternut Squash Risotto

Prep Time: 35 Minutes

Cook Time: 1hrs 30 Minutes

Servings: 2

Ingredients

- 1 1/2 lb. butternut squash
- 2 tsp. olive oil
- 1 large onion (finely diced)
- 1/2 cup arborio rice
- 3 cups water
- 1/4 tsp. salt
- ground black pepper to taste
- 6 ounces salmon (cut into thin strips)
- 2 ounces semi-soft goat cheese
- 1 Tbsp fresh oregano

Instructions

1   Preheat the oven to 325°F.
2   Cut the butternut squash in half lengthwise.
3   Scoop out the seeds and discard them.

4   Place 1 teaspoon olive oil in a small roasting pan.

5   Place the butternut squash in the pan cut side down and move around the pan to coat with the olive oil.

6   Put the pan in the oven and roast for 40 minutes.

7   Remove and let cool.

8   Cut half of the squash's flesh into about 1/2 inch dice, discarding the skin. (Reserve half of the butternut squash for another use.)

9   Place the remaining teaspoon olive oil in a skillet over medium high heat.

10 Add the onion when the oil is hot and cook for about 4 minutes. Stir frequently.

11 Add the rice.

12 Cook for about one minute. Stir continuously.

13 Add the water and salt. Stir, and when the water begins to boil, adjust the heat until the rice is simmering.

14 Simmer for about 20 minutes. Stir about once a minute.

15 Check the rice frequently for doneness. Add water two tablespoons at a time if extra water is needed.

16 When the rice is firm and not too soft - but not grainy - add the butternut squash, goat cheese, and the salmon.

17 Fold the fish and squash into the rice gently and cook for another 5 to 7 minutes until the cheese is melted and the salmon is done.

18 Add the oregano and gently fold into the rice.

19 Serve.

Prep Time: 45 Minutes

Cook Time: 2hrs 30 Minutes

Servings: 4

Ingredients

- 1 tsp. olive oil
- 1 large onion (diced)
- 3 cloves garlic (minced)
- 1/2 large green bell pepper (diced)
- 2 ribs celery (diced)
- 4 ounces spicy sausage (cut into 1/ inch cubes)
- 4 cups water
- 2 15-ounce cans no salt added kidney beans (drained and rinsed)
- 1 tsp. dried thyme leaves
- 3 tsp. salt free Creole Seasoning
- 1/4 tsp. salt
- fresh ground black pepper to taste
- 1/2 tsp. Tabasco Sauce
- 3 cups water
- 1 cup brown rice

Instructions

1   Place the oil in a large pan over medium heat.

2   Add the diced onions and garlic.

3   Cook for about five minutes. Stir frequently.

4   Add the celery and green pepper and cook, stirring frequently, for about 3 minutes.

5   Add the sausage and cook for about five minutes. Stir frequently.

6   Add the beans to the pot and then add the water, thyme leaves, Creole Seasoning, pepper, and Tabasco sauce.

7   Stir and reduce the heat to medium-low. Cook for about 2 hours, stirring occasionally. Add water about a half cup at a time as needed.

8   As the beans are nearly done (they should be soft and creamy) place the 3 cups water in a medium sauce pan over high heat.

9   When the water is boiling, add the rice, stir once, and reduce the heat to medium-low.

10 Cook, partially covered, until all the water is gone (35-45 minutes).

11 Stir the rice once to fluff it and then serve the red beans over the rice in 4 equal portions.

Prep Time: 10 Minutes

Cook Time: 30 Minutes

Servings: 4

Ingredients

- 1/2 cup reduced-fat (lite) unsweetened coconut milk
- 2 cloves garlic (minced)
- 2 Tbsp fresh lime juice
- 1 Tbsp fresh ginger (peeled and minced)
- 1 Tbsp low-sodium soy sauce orr gluten-free tamari sauce
- 1 tsp hoisin sauce or gluten-free hoisin sauce
- 1 Tbsp pure maple syrup
- 1 cup Thai or sweet basil (finely chopped)
- ounces large shrimp (peeled and deveined)

Instructions

1 Place the low-fat coconut milk, minced garlic, lime juice, minced ginger, low-sodium soy sauce, maple syrup and basil in a blender and puree until smooth.

2   Put the shrimp in a zipper bag and add the marinade.

3   Seal tightly and place in the refrigerator for at least 3 hours (overnight is best). Turn the bag from time to time to redistribute the marinade.

4   When ready to cook, preheat the oven to 400°F.

5   Place a large skillet in the oven and let heat for at least 10 minutes.

6   Add the marinated shrimp to the skillet.

7   As they sear on one side, top the other with about half of the marinade.

8   The shrimp will grill fast and should be turned after about three minutes.

9   Spread the remaining marinade over the top of the shrimp and grill for another 4 – 5 minutes.

10 Serve over Coconut Rice with 2 tablespoons of Thai Peanut Sauce.

Prep Time: 15 Minutes

Cook Time: 40 Minutes

Servings: 2

Ingredients

- 1 slice whole wheat or gluten free bread
- 1/2 tsp. dried oregano
- 1/2 tsp. dried basil
- 1/8 tsp. dried tarragon
- 1/4 tsp. dried marjoram
- to taste fresh ground black pepper
- 1 large egg
- 2 Tbsp. all purpose flour or garbanzo flour
- 2 tsp. unsalted butter
- 2 - 4 ounce boneless, skinless chicken breasts
- 1 ounce Parmigiano-Reggiano (grated)
- 6 Tbsp. **tomato sauce (or Low-Acid Tomato Sauce)**
- 2 ounces low-moisture mozzarella (shredded)

Instructions

1   Place the whole wheat bread in the oven and set the
    temperature to 300°F.
2   When the oven reaches 300° remove the bread and
    allow to sit for about 10 minutes.
3   Place a large skillet in the oven and increase the heat
    to 375°F.
4   Crumble the bread and place it in a mini chopper or
    blender with the oregano, basil, tarragon, marjoram,
    and pepper.
5   Process until the toast becomes coarse bread crumbs.
6   In a small bowl, whisk the egg until frothy.
7   Dip the chicken breasts in the flour (or garbanzo
    flour), then the egg to coat well, and then the
    seasoned bread crumbs.
8   Coat the chicken well, patting the bread crumbs in
    place.
9   Add the butter to the skillet.
10 Place the breaded chicken breasts in the pan.
11 Return the pan to the oven and cook for 12 minutes.
12 Turn the chicken breasts over and top with the grated
    parmesan (half over each chicken breast).
13 Cook for two minutes and top each chicken breast
    with three tablespoons of tomato sauce.

14 Place 1 ounce of the mozzarella cheese on top of each
    chicken breast and return the pan to the oven for
    about 2 - 3 minutes until the cheese is just melted.

15 Serve immediately.

Prep Time: 15 Minutes

Cook Time: 30 Minutes

Servings: 2

Ingredients

- 3 quarts water
- 2 large eggs
- 4 ounces whole wheat or gluten free rotini
- 2 tsp. olive oil
- 2 cloves garlic (minced)
- 2 ounces prosciutto (diced)
- 1 medium onion (diced)
- 1 cup frozen peas (thawed)
- 1 ounce parmesan (grated)
- fresh ground black pepper to taste

Instructions

1. Place the water in a large sauce pan over high heat.
2. When the water boils, add the eggs.

3   Cook for three minutes and then remove from the heat.

4   Let the eggs stand for 12 minutes in the hot water and then remove the eggs to a bowl of ice water.

5   Place the pan with the water back on the burner over high heat.

6   When the water boils again, add the rotini.

7   Cook for about 12 to 15 minutes until the pasta is just tender.

8   Drain the pasta.

9   While the pasta is cooking, place the olive oil in a large skillet over medium high heat.

10 Add the garlic and cook for one minute. Stir frequently.

11 Add the prosciutto and cook for about 2 minutes. Stir frequently.

12 Add the onion and cook for 7 to 10 minutes until the onion is translucent.

13 Adjust the heat to keep the onions from browning.

14 Place the onion and ham mixture in a large mixing bowl.

15 Add the peas and the cooked pasta.

16 Fold together gently.

17 Chill well.

18 When ready to serve, coarsely chop the hard-boiled
    eggs and add them to the salad with the parmesan and
    pepper.

19 Fold together gently and serve.

Prep Time: 15 Minutes

Cook Time: 45 Minutes

Servings: 2

Ingredients

- 2 – 4 ounce boneless pork chops
- 1 large egg
- 1 Tbsp. all purpose flour or garbanzo flour
- 1/3 cup panko crumbs or gluten-free panko crumbs
- black pepper to taste
- 1 Tbsp. olive oil (divided)

Instructions

1. Place the pork chops between two sheets of plastic wrap.
2. Using a meat mallet or a small sauce pan, pound the pork chops until about 1/2 inch thick. The pork chops should be uniformly thick.
3. Place the egg in a small bowl and whisk until smooth.
4. Place the flour in another small bowl.

5   Place the panko crumbs and pepper in a third small
    bowl and whisk with a fork to combine.

6   Dredge the pork chop in the flour to coat completely.

7   Immediately dredge the coated pork chop in the egg
    to coat completely.

8   Immediately dredge the coated pork chop in the
    panko crumbs to coat completely. As you coat the
    panko crumbs on the pork chop, press gently to help
    the panko to stick. Repeat for each pork chop.

9   Place a large skillet over medium high heat.

10 Add one teaspoon of the olive oil and then gently
    place the pork chops in the pan.

11 Cook for about 8 minutes. Adjust the heat so the
    breadcrumbs brown lightly but do not burn.

12 Add a teaspoon of olive oil and turn. Cook for another
    6 to 8 minutes.

13 Add another teaspoon of oil and turn the pork chop.
    Cook for another 3 to 4 minutes.

14 Serve topped with **Ranch Dressing.**

Prep Time: 10 Minutes

Cook Time: 50 Minutes

Servings: 2

Ingredients

- 2 1/2 cups water
- 1/2 cup brown rice
- 4 large green onions
- 2 tsp. sesame oil
- 2 Tbsp. fresh ginger root (peeled and minced)
- 1 large carrots (peeled and diced)
- 1 rib celery (diced)
- 6 ounces pork chop (cut into 1/2 inch dice)
- fresh ground black pepper to taste
- 4 tsp. low sodium soy sauce or gluten-free tamari sauce
- 2 tsp. Dijon or Chinese mustard
- 1/2 tsp. honey
- 1/2 tsp. five spice powder
- 1 cup vegetable stock
- 2/3 cup frozen peas (thawed)

- 2 large eggs (beaten)

Instructions

1. Place the water in a small sauce pan over high heat.
2. When the water boils, add the rice and reduce the heat to a simmer.
3. Cook, partially covered, until the water cooks away. Do not stir the rice. When cooked, remove from the stove and set aside.
4. Cut the white bottoms off of the green onions. Slice the white part crosswise into 1/2 inch lengths.
5. Cut the green tops crosswise into 1/4 inch slices.
6. When ready to cook place the sesame oil in a wok or large skillet over high heat.
7. Add the ginger and the carrots and cook for 2 to 4 minutes. Stir frequently.
8. Add the celery. Cook for about 3 minutes. Stir frequently.
9. Add the pork and the white part of the green onions and cook until the pork begins to brown. Stir frequently.

10 Place the soy sauce, mustard, honey, five spice powder
    and vegetable stock in a small bowl and whisk until
    blended.

11 Add the rice and sauce to the vegetables in the skillet.

12 Cook for about 3 minutes. Stir frequently.

13 Add the peas and the green tops of the green onions.
    Stir well.

14 Add the beaten eggs and toss until the egg is cooked
    through.

15 Serve.

19. Blue Cheese Crab Cakes

Prep Time: 10 Minutes

Cook Time: 30 Minutes

Servings: 4

Ingredients

- 8 ounces lump crabmeat
- 1 tsp. Dijon mustard
- 1 large egg
- 1 Tbsp. fresh lemon juice
- 1 ounce blue cheese
- 1/4 cup whole wheat or gluten free breadcrumbs
- 1 Tbsp. shallot (minced)
- 1 small rib celery (diced)
- fresh ground black pepper to taste
- 2 tsp. extra virgin olive oil

Instructions

1. Pick over crabmeat, removing any shell.
2. Place in a medium mixing bowl.

3 Place the mustard, egg, lemon juice, and blue cheese in a blender or mini chopper.

4 Process until smooth.

5 Add the breadcrumbs, shallot, celery, and blue cheese mixture to the mixing bowl with the crab.

6 Season with pepper.

7 Fold together gently until well blended. Be careful to not break up the crabmeat too much.

8 Form into 4 cakes and chill. These can be made up to 12 hours in advance.

9 Preheat the oven to 400° F.

10 Place the oil in a large skillet over high heat until the oil is almost smoking.

11 Place cakes in the hot oil to cook and reduce the heat to medium-high.

12 Cook for about three minutes.

13 Turn the cakes over and cook for about 2 minutes.

14 Place the pan in the hot oven.

15 Cook for another 9 – 10 minutes.

20. Risotto Con Camarones (Shrimp)

Prep Time: 10 Minutes

Cook Time: 30 Minutes

Servings: 4

Ingredients

- 2 tsp. olive oil
- 2 Tbsp. pumpkin seeds
- 2 cloves garlic (minced)
- 1 medium red onion (diced)
- 1/2 cup arborio rice
- 3 1/2 cups water
- 1 tsp. paprika
- 1/8 tsp. saffron
- 1/4 tsp. ground cumin
- 1/4 tsp. salt
- fresh ground black pepper to taste
- 8 grape tomatoes
- 8 ounces shrimp (peeled, deveined, and sliced in half lengthwise)
- 1/4 cup frozen peas (thawed and rinsed)
- 1 ounce semi soft goat cheese

- 1/2 medium red bell pepper (diced)
- 1/2 medium yellow bell pepper (diced)
- 2 Tbsp. fresh cilantro leaves (coarsely chopped)

Instructions

1. Heat 1 teaspoon of the olive oil in a medium sized non-stock skillet over medium heat.
2. Add the pumpkin seeds and cook, stirring frequently, until they begin to turn brown.
3. Add the garlic and cook for about one minute.
4. Add the diced onion and cook, stirring frequently, for about 5 minutes.
5. Add the arborio and stir it into the onions for about a minute.
6. Add the water, paprika, saffron, cumin, salt and pepper.
7. Cook over medium heat. Stir frequently.
8. As the rice nears being done place a large skillet over medium heat.
9. Add 1 teaspoon olive oil and add the tomatoes.
10. Cook for 5 minutes. Stir frequently.
11. While the tomatoes are cooking add the shrimp, peas, and the goat cheese to the risotto.
12. Fold together gently while the shrimp cooks and the cheese melts.
13. While the shrimp is cooking, add the diced yellow and red pepper to the pan with the tomatoes.
14. Cook for about 3 - 5 minutes, stirring frequently.

15 When the risotto is done, serve topped with the tomatoes and peppers.

16 Sprinkle the cilantro over the top and serve.

DINNERS

21. Lemon Shrimp Quinoa Salad

Prep Time: 10 Minutes

Cook Time: 1hrs 10 Minutes

Servings: 4

Ingredients

- ounces shrimp (peeled and deveined)
- 1 lemon (zested and juiced)
- 1 - 15 ounce can no salt added chickpeas (drained and rinsed)
- 3 tsp. olive oil (divided)
- 4 cloves garlic (minced)
- 1 medium red onion (finely diced)
- 1 cup no salt added vegetable stock
- 1/2 cup water
- 1 orange (zested and juiced)
- 1 cup quinoa
- 1/2 tsp. salt
- black pepper to taste

- 1/4 cup white wine
- 1 cucumber (diced)
- 8 ounces grape or cherry tomatoes (halved)
- 1 Tbsp. fresh dill
- 2 ounces feta cheese (crumbled)

Instructions

1   Place the shrimp in a bowl with the lemon juice and the lemon zest.

2   Toss well and set aside.

3   Place the drained chickpeas in a large mixing bowl and set aside.

4   Place a large skillet over medium high heat.

5   Add two teaspoons of the olive oil, and when it is hot, add the garlic.

6   Cook for about one minute, then add the onion.

7   Cook for about 4 minutes. Stir frequently and adjust the heat so the onions are translucent but still slightly firm.

8   Add the vegetable stock, water, orange juice, orange zest, quinoa, salt, and pepper.

9   When the liquid comes to a boil, reduce the heat, cover, and let simmer for 15 minutes.

10 Remove from the heat and let stand for 5 minutes.

11 While the quinoa is cooking, place a second large skillet over medium high heat.

12 Add 1 teaspoon of the olive oil and then the shrimp.

13 Saute for about 4 minutes on one side and turn the shrimp.

14 Cook for another 4 minutes and place the shrimp in the bowl with the chickpeas.

15 Add the remaining liquid from the marinade and the white wine to the pan.

16 Cook until the wine is reduced to about 2 tablespoons, scraping the bottom of the pan frequently.

17 Add the liquid to the bowl with the chickpeas and shrimp.

18 When the quinoa is done cooking and resting, add the quinoa to the bowl with the chickpeas and shrimp.

19 Chill well.

20 When the salad is cold, add the cucumber, tomato, dill, and feta cheese.

21 Fold together gently and serve.

Prep Time: 10 Minutes

Cook Time: 1hrs 10 Minutes

Servings: 4

Ingredients

- 8 quarts water
- 1 medium spaghetti squash (about 2 lbs)
- 4 tsp. olive oil
- 2 medium onion (diced)
- 4 Tbsp. all-purpose flour or garbanzo flour
- 1 tsp. curry powder
- 1 tsp. garam masala
- 1/2 tsp. cumin
- 1/4 tsp. cayenne
- 2 cups no salt added vegetable stock
- 1 cup lite coconut milk
- 1/2 tsp. salt
- oz. shrimp (peeled and deveined)
- 2 oz. semi-soft goat cheese
- large leaves fresh basil (chiffonade)
- 4 ounces roasted, unsalted cashews (roughly chopped)

Instructions

1. Place the spaghetti squash in a large stockpot and cover with water. Bring to a boil and reduce heat to simmer.

2. Simmer, partially covered, for about 40 minutes.

3. Remove the squash. When the squash is cool enough to handle, slice the squash lengthwise. Using a spoon, scrape out the seeds from each half and discard.

4. Using a fork, scrape the spaghetti squash strands into a bowl, separating the strands into spaghetti-like strands. Set aside. (Consider placing the shredded strands in an oven set to "warm" or about 170F until needed.)

5. Place the olive oil in a large saucepan over medium-high heat.

6. Add the onions and cook, stirring frequently, for 10 minutes, adjusting the heat so that the onions are no more than lightly browned. (Note that this sauce should never boil or even simmer throughout cooking.)

7. Add the curry powder, garam masala, cumin, and cayenne, and cook, stirring constantly, for about 2 minutes.

8   Add the flour or garbanzo flour and cook, stirring constantly, until just blended - about 30-60 seconds.

9   Add the vegetable stock and salt and stir until the sauce begins to thicken.

10 Add the coconut milk, stir thoroughly, and cook for another 5-7 minutes until the sauce thickens more.

11 Add the shrimps and goat cheese and cook, stirring gently and occasionally, until the shrimps are cooked through and the goat cheese is melted: 7-10 minutes.

12 Divide the spaghetti squash among four plates and top with equal amounts of the shrimp and sauce. Sprinkle the cashews and basil over the top and serve.

Prep Time: 30 Minutes

Cook Time: 1hrs 25 Minutes

Servings: 4

Ingredients

- 1 tsp. olive oil
- 1 medium onion (diced)
- 1 large carrot (peeled and cut into small dice)
- 1 medium red bell pepper (diced)
- 1 Tbsp. chili powder
- 1/2 tsp. ground cumin
- 1 Tbsp. smoked paprika
- 1 tsp. dried oregano
- 1/2 tsp. salt
- 2 – 15 ounce cans no salt added diced tomatoes
- 2 – 15 ounce cans no salt added white beans (drained and rinsed)
- 2 cups no salt added vegetable stock
- 1 medium zucchini (diced)
- 1 ear corn (shuck kernels from cob) or 1 cup frozen corn

- 4 Tbsp. reduced fat sour cream
- 2 ounces reduced fat cheddar cheese

Instructions

1. Place the oil in a large sauce pan over medium high heat.
2. Add the onion and carrot and cook for about 5 to 7 minutes. Stir frequently.
3. Add the red bell pepper and cook for about 3 minutes. Stir frequently.
4. Add the chili powder, cumin, paprika, oregano, salt, tomatoes, white beans, and vegetable stock.
5. Stir and reduce the heat to medium low and simmer for 20 minutes.
6. Add the zucchini and corn.
7. Simmer for another 10 minutes. Stir occasionally.
8. Serve topped with the sour cream and cheddar cheese.

Prep Time: 30 Minutes

Cook Time: 1hrs 25 Minutes

Servings: 4

Ingredients

- 2 tsp. olive oil
- 1 large onion (sliced)
- ounces carrots (peeled and cut into 1/2 inch cubes)
- 2 15-ounce cans no salt added garbanzo beans
- 2 15-ounce cans no salt added diced tomatoes
- 2 cups no salt added vegetable stock
- 2 cups water
- 1/4 cup white wine
- 1 tsp. ground cinnamon
- 1 tsp. ground cumin
- 2 tsp. paprika
- 1/2 tsp. red pepper flakes
- 1 tsp. ground coriander
- 1/4 tsp. salt
- large green olives (sliced)
- 1/2 cup lentils

- 1/2 cup non-fat Greek yogurt
- 2 Tbsp. harissa sauce

Instructions

1. Place the olive oil in a large stock pot or dutch oven over medium high heat.
2. When the oil is hot, add the onions. Cook for about 4 minutes. Stir frequently.
3. Add the carrots, garbanzo beans, tomatoes, vegetable stock, water, wine, cinnamon, cumin, paprika, red pepper flakes, coriander, and salt.
4. Stir, reduce the heat to medium and cover.
5. Simmer for 1 hour. Stir occasionally.
6. After the first hour add the olives and stir.
7. Cook for 10 minutes and add the lentils. Stir.
8. Cook for 20 minutes. Stir occasionally.
9. Combine the yogurt and harissa sauce in a small bowl and stir gently until well blended.
10. Serve the stew topped with the yogurt sauce.

Prep Time: 20 Minutes

Cook Time: 1hrs 35 Minutes

Servings: 4

Ingredients

- 1 ounce dried mushrooms (porcini or portobello)
- 2 cups boiling water
- 2 tsp. olive oil
- 1 large onion (thinly sliced)
- ounces crimini mushrooms (cut into quarters)
- 2 cups vegetable stock
- 2 cups water
- 2 large carrots (peeled and cut into 1/2 inch chunks
- ounces red or Yukon Gold potatoes (cut into 1/2 inch chunks)
- 1/2 tsp. salt
- black pepper to taste
- 1 Tbsp. dried sage
- 1 tsp. dried marjoram
- 2 Tbsp. Worcestershire sauce
- 8 ounces shallots (peeled and left whole)

- 1/4 cup red table wine

Instructions

1. Place the dried mushrooms in a large bowl and pour the boiling water over the top.
2. Stir gently and let stand.
3. Place the olive oil in a large sauce pan or small stock pot over high heat.
4. Add the onion and cook for about 3 minutes. Stir frequently.
5. Add the crimini mushrooms and continue to cook over high heat. Stir frequently.
6. Cook for about 10 minutes, until the mushrooms brown.
7. Add the vegetable stock, water, carrots, potatoes, salt, pepper, sage, marjoram, and Worcestershire sauce.
8. Stir and reduce the heat until the stew is simmering.
9. Strain the liquid from the dried mushrooms into the pot and stir.
10. Coarsely chop the reconstituted dried mushrooms and add to the pot.
11. Simmer for 30 minutes. Stir occasionally.
12. Add the shallots and wine.

13 Stir and simmer for another 30 minutes, stirring
    occasionally.
14 Serve.

Prep Time: 10 Minutes

Cook Time: 35 Minutes

Servings: 4

Ingredients

- 3 quarts water
- 8 ounces whole wheat or gluten free pasta
- 2 tsp. olive oil
- 2 cloves garlic (minced)
- 1 bunch collard greens (about 3 cups)(thinly sliced crosswise)
- 1/4 tsp. dried thyme
- 1 15-ounce can no salt added white beans (drained and rinsed)
- 1/2 tsp. salt
- black pepper to taste
- 1/2 cup white wine
- 1/2 lemon (juiced)
- 1 1/2 ounces parmesan cheese (grated)

Instructions

1. Place the water in a large pot over high heat.
2. When the water boils, add the pasta.
3. Stir and boil for about 12 to 15 minutes until al dente.
4. While the pasta is cooking, place the olive oil in a large skillet over medium heat.
5. Add the garlic and cook for about one minute. Stir frequently.
6. Add the collard greens and cook for about two minutes until just wilted. Toss frequently.
7. Add the thyme, white beans, salt, pepper, white wine, and lemon juice.
8. Stir and cook for about 1 minute. Toss frequently.
9. When the pasta is done, drain and add to the greens with the parmesan cheese.
10. Toss well and serve.

Prep Time: 15 Minutes

Cook Time: 1hrs 15 Minutes

Servings: 2

Ingredients

- 2 lb. spaghetti squash (sliced in half lengthwise and seeded)
- 2 tsp. olive oil
- 1/2 large onion (diced)
- 2 cloves garlic (minced)
- 1 15-ounce can no salt added diced tomatoes
- 1/4 tsp. salt
- black pepper to taste
- 1 tsp. dried basil
- 1/2 tsp. dried oregano
- 1/4 tsp. dried marjoram
- 1 15-ounce can no salt added white beans (drained and rinsed)
- 3 Tbsp. parsley (coarsely chopped)
- 1 ounce parmesan cheese (grated)

Instructions

1 Preheat the oven to 350°F.

2 Place 1 teaspoon of the olive oil in a large skillet or on a baking sheet.

3 Place the squash in the pan cut side down and place the pan in the oven.

4 Roast for 45 minutes.

5 When the squash is tender, remove from the oven and set aside to cool.

6 When the squash is cool enough to handle, use a fork to gently remove the flesh of the squash in strands.

7 Place 1 teaspoon olive oil in a large skillet over medium high heat.

8 Add the onion and cook for 4 to 5 minutes. Stir frequently.

9 Add the garlic and cook for one minute. Stir frequently.

10 Add the tomatoes, salt, pepper, basil, oregano, and marjoram.

11 Stir and cover the pan.

12 Simmer over medium low heat for 20 minutes. Stir occasionally.

13 Add the white beans to the pan.

14 Stir and cook for another 5 minutes.

15 Add the spaghetti squash to the tomato sauce with the
    parsley and parmesan.
16 Stir gently and heat through.
17 Serve.

Prep Time: 15 Minutes

Cook Time: 1hrs 15 Minutes

Servings: 2

Ingredients

- 2 tsp. olive oil (divided)
- 1 1/4 large onion (diced)
- 8 ounces crimini mushrooms (diced)
- 1 1/2 tsp. chili powder
- 1 1/2 tsp. smoked paprika
- 1/2 tsp. ground cumin
- ounces fresh spinach
- 6 ounces tomatillos (coarsely chopped)
- 1 ounce goat cheese
- 6 corn tortillas
- 3 ounces reduced fat Monterey jack cheese (grated)
- 4 Tbsp. fresh cilantro leaves

Instructions

1. Place one teaspoon of the olive oil in a large skillet over medium high heat.
2. Add the diced 1 large onion and sauté for about 5 minutes.
3. Add the mushrooms and cook for about 5 to 7 minutes. Stir frequently.
4. Add the chili powder, paprika, and cumin.
5. Cook for about one minute until the spices are well blended.
6. Add the spinach and cook until it is wilted. Toss frequently.
7. Remove the spinach and mushroom mixture from the pan and set aside to cool.
8. While the spinach is cooling, add the remaining 1 teaspoon olive oil and the 1/4 large diced onion.
9. Cook for about 5 minutes. Stir frequently.
10. Add the tomatillos and reduce the heat to medium.
11. Cook for 15 minutes.
12. Let cool slightly and then place in a blender with the goat cheese.
13. Puree until smooth.
14. When ready to serve, preheat the oven to broil.
15. Reheat the spinach mixture and the tomatillo sauce.

16 Evenly divide the spinach mixture between the corn tortillas and roll into a cigar shape.

17 Place three of the tortillas each in an oven proof bowl.

18 Top with the tomatillo sauce and then the jack cheese.

19 Place the bowls under the broiler and cook until the cheese melts and browns lightly.

20 Serve topped with the fresh cilantro.

29. Pinto Bean and Butternut Squash Quesadilla

Prep Time: 30 Minutes

Cook Time: 1hrs 20 Minutes

Servings: 4

Ingredients

- 1 lb. butternut squash
- 1/2 cup 2% milk
- 2 tsp. olive oil
- 2 cloves garlic (minced)
- 1 15-ounce can no salt added pinto beans (drained and rinsed)
- 1 tsp. ground cumin
- 1 tsp. smoked paprika
- 1/2 tsp. chili powder
- 1/2 tsp. dried oregano
- 1/4 tsp. salt
- ground black pepper to taste
- 1/2 cup water
- spray olive oil
- 2 Tbsp. fresh cilantro (chopped)
- 1/2 cup pumpkin seeds

- 8 6-inch corn tortillas

- 6 ounces reduced fat Monterey jack cheese (grated)

- 4 Tbsp. reduced fat sour cream

Instructions

1 Preheat the oven to 325°F.

2 Cut the butternut squash in half lengthwise.

3 Scoop out the seeds and discard them.

4 Place 1 teaspoon olive oil in a small roasting pan.

5 Place the butternut squash in the pan cut side down and move around the pan to coat with the olive oil.

6 Put the pan in the oven and roast for 40 minutes.

7 Remove and let cool.

8 Peel the squash and cut into about 1/2 inch dice. (Reserve half of the butternut squash for another use.)

9 Place the squash in a blender with the milk and puree until smooth.

10 Place the olive oil in a skillet over medium high heat.

11 Add the garlic when the oil is hot and cook for about 1 minute. Stir frequently.

12 Add the beans.

13 Cook for about one minute. Stir continuously.

14 Add the cumin, paprika, chili powder, oregano, salt, pepper and water.

15 Stir and when the water begins to boil adjust the heat until it is simmering.

16 Simmer for about 5 minutes. Stir occasionally.

17 Stir in the butternut squash puree and the cilantro and 1/4 cup of the pumpkin seeds.

18 Place a large skillet or griddle over high heat. When hot spray with oil.

19 Add four corn tortillas and then top each with 1/4 of the bean and butternut squash mixture.

20 Top with the cheese and then each with another corn tortilla.

21 Lightly spray the top of the quesadillas with oil.

22 Cook for about 5 minutes on the first side, turn and cook for another 4 to 5 minutes.

23 Serve topped with 1 tablespoon of sour cream and 1 tablespoon of pumpkin seeds per quesadilla.

Prep Time: 10 Minutes

Cook Time: 30 Minutes

Servings: 2

Ingredients

- 4 quarts water
- 4 ounces whole wheat or gluten-free elbow pasta
- 1 large egg
- 1/4 cup 2% milk (1 % milk will work)
- 2 1/2 ounces reduced-fat cheddar cheese (grated)
- 1/8 tsp salt
- fresh ground black pepper to taste

Instructions

1. Place the water in a medium stock-pot over high heat and bring to a boil. Add the pasta and cook until done. Do not overcook - the pasta should be cooked al dente.

2   While the pasta is cooking, combine the eggs and milk in a medium sauce pan. Whisk until smooth. Add the reduced-fat cheddar cheese and salt.

3   When the pasta is done, drain well and add it to the pot with the cheese over medium heat. Stir well until the cheese is completely melted and creamy. Don't let the mixture boil, and when the sauce is very thick, remove from the heat.

4   Add fresh ground black pepper to taste, stir, and serve immediately.